Jéssica Ribeiro Magalhães
Andréia V. C. Amaral

Glaucoma induced by iatrogenic hyperadrenocorticism

Jéssica Ribeiro Magalhães
Andréia V. C. Amaral

Glaucoma induced by iatrogenic hyperadrenocorticism

Case report

Imprint

Any brand names and product names mentioned in this book are subject to trademark, brand or patent protection and are trademarks or registered trademarks of their respective holders. The use of brand names, product names, common names, trade names, product descriptions etc. even without a particular marking in this work is in no way to be construed to mean that such names may be regarded as unrestricted in respect of trademark and brand protection legislation and could thus be used by anyone.

Cover image: www.ingimage.com

This book is a translation from the original published under ISBN 978-613-9-74616-3.

Publisher:
Sciencia Scripts
is a trademark of
Dodo Books Indian Ocean Ltd. and OmniScriptum S.R.L publishing group

120 High Road, East Finchley, London, N2 9ED, United Kingdom
Str. Armeneasca 28/1, office 1, Chisinau MD-2012, Republic of Moldova, Europe
Printed at: see last page
ISBN: 978-620-6-31526-1

I dedicate this work to my parents, my sister, and my boyfriend for their support and affection.

ACKNOWLEDGEMENTS

I thank God for granting life.

I thank my parents, André Luiz Magalhães de Oliveira Lima and Sueli Carvalho Ribeiro Magalhães, who taught me everything I know today. Thank you for your love, affection, understanding, respect, education. Without you I would not have my foundation in life.

To my sister Joyce Ribeiro Magalhães, for always being by my side, for her care and love.

To my boyfriend Leandro Silva Onofre Junior, for being by my side at all times, for his encouragement and affection.

I thank the advisor Prof.ª Dr³ . Andréia Vitor Couto do Amaral, for her dedication and attention. For always being willing to help in the intellectual enrichment of each of her students.

I also thank the team of the Veterinary Hospital of UFG, Campus Jataí. With you I have learnt how a good professional can make a difference.

To all, my sincere thanks!

SUMMARY

SUMMARY

Hyperadrenocorticism (HAC) or *Cushing*'s Syndrome is a common endocrinopathy in adult and aged dogs, which induces clinical changes due to glucocorticoid excess and can be endogenous or exogenous (iatrogenic). Iatrogenic CAH is manifested by a variety of symptoms. Dogs affected by the syndrome may present with hypertension, which can lead to numerous lesions in target organs such as the eyes, kidneys, brain and cardiovascular system. In the eyes, CAH may lead to hypertensive retinopathy. Glaucoma, secondary to hypertensive retinopathy, is characterised by progressive loss of visual function, apoptosis and death of retinal ganglion cells and their axons, and blindness. Impairment of the balance between aqueous humour production and drainage can result in variations in intraocular pressure that trigger glaucoma. The present report describes glaucoma secondary to iatrogenic *Cushing*'s syndrome in a dog.

Keywords: dog, corticosteroids, hypertension, retinopathy.

CHAPTER 1

1. INTRODUCTION

Hyperadrenocorticism (HAC) or *Cushing*'s Syndrome is a disorder that is associated with excessive rates of endogenous or exogenous glucocorticoids. This endocrinopathy can occur endogenously or exogenously (iatrogenic). Its endogenous form may have pituitary or pituitary-dependent origin and adrenocortical or adrenal-dependent neoplastic origin (AIELLO, 2001).

Pituitary-dependent CAH accounts for 80 to 85% of cases, while adrenal-dependent CAH occurs in about 15 to 20% of cases (AIELLO, 2001).

On the other hand, iatrogenic CAH is due to the chronic administration of glucocorticoids, which are usually used to control hypersensitivity disorders or immune-mediated diseases, and corresponds to the most frequent type in dogs (ABREU, 2012).

The clinical signs of the different types of CAH result from the combination of gluconeogenic, lipolytic, anti-inflammatory, immunosuppressive and protein catabolic effects of glucocorticoids (LEAL, 2008).

The commonly observed complications resulting from HAC are Diabetes *Mellitus*, lower urinary tract infections, tachypnoea, bronchopneumonia and pulmonary thromboembolism, in addition to hypertension that affects several body systems (LOPES, 2011).

More than half of dogs with CAH are hypertensive. Due to hypertension, many dogs with this syndrome may develop ophthalmological changes, such as increased intraocular pressure (IOP), retinal detachment or intraocular haemorrhage, which can lead to glaucoma or blindness (LEAL, 2008).

Glaucoma is currently considered the final pathway of diseases characterised by progressive loss of sensitivity and function, apoptosis and death of retinal ganglion cells and their axons, and blindness (MARTINS et al., 2006).

Clinical signs in glaucoma may vary according to the stage of glaucoma. Conjunctival hyperaemia, engorged episcleral vessels, corneal oedema and ulceration, lens dislocation, buftalmia and fractures of the *Descemet's* membrane are commonly observed (MARTINS et al., 2006).

The case presented shows how erroneous glucocorticoid medication can trigger systemic metabolic changes in a dog, among which is glaucoma with consequent complete loss of visual function.

CHAPTER 2

2.   HYPERADRENOCORTICISM OR *CUSHING'S* SYNDROME

Hyperadrenocorticism (HAC) or Cushing's Syndrome is a disorder of circulating cortisol levels. It has no sex predisposition but is common in adult to elderly dogs and rare in cats (FELDMAN, 2012).

2.1. Pathophysiology

2.1.1. Pituitary or pituitary-dependent hyperadrenocorticism

It is the most common endogenous form (ABREU, 2012). The presence of tumours or pituitary hyperplasia increases the secretion of adrenocorticotropic hormone (ACTH) which results in bilateral adrenocortical hyperplasia and excess cortisol production. This excess leads to failure of the negative *feedback* mechanism on ACTH (NELSON & COUTO, 2006).

2.1.2. Adrenal-dependent hyperadrenocorticism or adrenal neoplasia

It is related to the presence of adrenal tumours. They are usually unilateral tumours (SCARAMPELLA, 2011). The adrenocortical tumour stimulates excessive cortisol production independent of pituitary control. The cortisol released inhibits the production of ACTH in the pituitary gland, but the adrenal tumour continues to release cortisol in a disorderly manner (TEIXEIRA, 2009).

2.1.3. Iatrogenic hyperadrenocorticism

It results from excessive administration of glucocorticoids that cause bilateral adrenocortical atrophy (NELSON & COUTO, 2006). It is the most common form of CAH in dogs (ABREU, 2012).

2.2. Epidemiology

The iatrogenic form of CAH is the most frequent in dogs, and has no age, sex or breed predisposition. It usually manifests in patients treated chronically with systemic corticosteroids (ABREU, 2012).

Pituitary-dependent CAH is more common in small breeds. Adrenal-dependent CAH, on the other hand, more often affects medium to large breeds (RAMSEY & RISTIC, 2007).

Cushing's Syndrome is a pathology mainly of adult to elderly animals between the ages of 6 and 16 (HÉRIPRET, 2008).

2.3. Clinical Signs

CAH has an insidious onset and progresses slowly (ABREU, 2012). Chronic exposure to excess cortisol can result in the development of a combination of drastic clinical signs. These signs include polydipsia, polyuria, polyphagia, increased abdominal volume (or obesity), alopecia (sparing the head and distal extremities), thin coat, hair growth failure, pyoderma, wheezing, hepatomegaly, muscle weakness, lethargy, calcinosis cutis, testicular atrophy, anestrus in females, heat intolerance, acne (skin infection, comedones), and skin hyperpigmentation. Not all animals with CAH develop the same clinical signs (LEAL, 2008).

The signs are the sequelae of the combined gluconeogenic, immunosuppressive, anti-inflammatory, protein catabolic and lipolytic effects of glucocorticoids on various organ systems (LEAL, 2008).

2.3.1. Dermatological signs

The first of the effects of glucocorticoids is the inhibition of keratinocyte proliferation leading to skin atrophy, wrinkling of the skin and excessive desquamation (OLIVEIRA, 2012).

The skin of dogs affected by CAH is thin, hypotonic, fragile, dry and with little elasticity (SCARAMPELLA, 2011; OLIVEIRA, 2012). It is also possible to observe hyperpigmentation of the skin, phlebectasia, seborrhoea (dry or oily), pyoderma and comedones (SCARAMPELLA, 2011).

2.3.2. Polyuria/Polydipsia

About 90% of dogs with CAH show these signs. Polyuria is possibly caused by glucocorticoids interfering with the action of antidiuretic hormone (ADH) in the renal tubules (KOOISTRA & GALAC, 2010; HERRTAGE, 2011).

2.3.3. Polyphagia

It occurs in the same proportion as polyuria and polydipsia (about 90% of dogs with CAH). It is related to the decreased concentration of corticotrophin-releasing hormone (CRH) and the anti-insulin effect of cortisol. The dog starts stealing food and rummaging through rubbish (CARVALHO, 2009).

2.3.4. Abdominal Distension

Abdominal distension is frequently observed in dogs with CAH. It arises due to increased adipose tissue in the abdomen and weakening and loss of muscle mass due to protein catabolism (HERRTAGE, 2011).

Hepatomegaly contributes to the increased abdominal volume and is easily palpable (FELDMAN, 2004).

2.3.5. Muscle changes

Weakness, muscle atrophy and lethargy are consequences of increased glucocorticoids that favour protein catabolism (ALENZA, 2011).

Dogs with CAH usually present tachypnoea due to reduced lung capacity due to loss of musculature and weakness of the muscles involved in breathing, in addition to the deposit of fat on the thorax (BIRCHARD & SHERDING, 2003).

2.3.6. Reproductive Signs

Anaestrus in females and testicular atrophy in males are caused by negative feedback from hypercortisolism, which result in a reduction in pituitary gonadotropin secretion (FELDMAN, 2004).

2.3.7. Neurological Signs

The growth and expansion of pituitary tumours can cause signs such as walking in circles, seizures, behavioural changes and stupor (BIRCHARD & SHERDING, 2003).

Lethargy is one of the main neurological signs presented by patients with CAH and may be associated with high ACTH concentration or the effects of excess cortisol on brain enzymes (BIRCHARD &

SHERDING, 2003).

2.3.8. Ophthalmological Signs

In cases of pituitary macroadenoma, the animal may present vision loss, facial paralysis and exophthalmos due to compression of structures adjacent to the neoplasm (GELLAT, 2007).

Infectious processes can trigger panuveitis and retinopathy. Retinal haemorrhages and detachments as well as hyphema may arise secondary to hypertension and consequent hypertensive retinopathy (LEAL, 2008).

Animals with CAH may present calcium deposits at the level of the corneal stroma, which together with ulcers may progress to corneal perforation. Hypertriglyceridaemia may also occur, predisposing to *retinal* lipaemia, lipaemic aqueous humour and lipid deposition in the cornea (LEAL, 2008).

More rarely, SARD (*Sudden Acquired Retinal Degeneration*), a non-inflammatory retinal syndrome resulting from degeneration and loss of photoreceptors, may occur, progressing to permanent blindness (ETTINGER & FELDMAN, 2010).

2.4. Diagnosis

The diagnosis of CAH should be based on clinical suspicion together with anamnesis, physical examination and laboratory tests (MASCHIETTO, 2007).

Clinicopathological studies such as haemogram, serum biochemistry and complete urinalysis with culture are of fundamental importance. ETTINGER & FELDMAN (2010) recommend abdominal ultrasound examination in addition to skin histology, computed tomography or magnetic resonance imaging.

Endocrine tests are essential in the diagnosis of CAH, however, they should only be used to confirm clinical suspicion of the disease (ETTINGER & FELDMAN, 2010).

2.4.1. Blood count

A "stress leucogram" is usually observed, with neutrophilia without left shift, monocytosis, lymphopenia and eosinopenia (LEAL, 2008; LIMA, 2008).

2.4.2. Serum Biochemistry

• Glucose: glycaemia is one of the most common alterations. It may be severely increased because glucocorticoids increase hepatic gluconeogenesis and decrease peripheral glucose utilisation by antagonising the effects of insulin (MICELI et al., 2012).

• Urea and Creatinine: increased urea concentration due to protein catabolism. Creatinine in 50% of cases may be below reference values due to excessive diuresis (LEAL, 2008).

• Liver enzymes: alanine aminotransferase (ALT) and alkaline phosphatase (ALP) will be increased in CAH. ALT increases as a result of hepatocyte lysis and glycogen accumulation (ALENZA, 2011; HERRTAGE, 2011). FA increases due to glucocorticoids inducing the production of the steroid-dependent alkaline phosphatase isoenzyme (s-PAI) by hepatocytes and bile duct endothelial cells. In addition, vacuolisation and glycogen overload secondary to the effects of glucocorticoids promote cholestasis responsible for increasing AF (LEAL, 2008; LIMA, 2008; SILVA, 2013).

• Cholesterol and triglycerides: lipolysis stimulated by glucocorticoids increases serum lipid and cholesterol concentrations (ALENZA, 2011).

2.4.3. . Urinalysis

Dogs with CAH have a urinary density of less than 1015. Isostenuria and hypostenuria are common and confirm polydipsia and polyuria (NELSON & COUTO, 2009).

Proteinuria can also occur and may be caused by glomerulopathies, systemic hypertension, or even the presence of lower urinary tract infection (UTI) (ETTINGER & FELDMAN, 2010; ALENZA, 2011).

UTI is not always diagnosed due to hypostenuria and the anti-inflammatory effects of glucocorticoids that usually interfere with the identification of inflammatory cells in urine (HERRTAGE, 2011).

2.4.4. . Abdominal ultrasound

The adrenals appear hypoechogenic in relation to the kidneys under anatomical conditions. To determine the dimensions, longitudinal, medial-lateral and ventro-dorsal measurements should be taken (LEAL, 2008).

If the adrenal glands are symmetrically enlarged, with no change in contour or echogenicity, there is a strong suspicion of pituitary-dependent hyperadrenocorticism, since bilateral adrenal tumours are rare (ETTINGER & FELDMAN, 2010).

2.4.5. Computerised Tomography and Magnetic Resonance Imaging

These tests are useful in assessing the size and symmetry of the pituitary and adrenal glands, as well as in identifying and assessing tumours present in them. They also assist in the selection of treatment (TAODA et al., 2011).

2.4.6. . Endocrine Tests

• ACTH Stimulation Test: Has moderate sensitivity and specificity (GILOR & GRAVES, 2011). Dogs with pituitary-dependent CAH or adrenal neoplasia show an exaggerated cortisol response after ACTH stimulation, whereas iatrogenic CAH shows no or decreased response after ACTH stimulation (FORD & MAZZAFERRO, 2007; FELDMAN, 2004). This test allows diagnosing hypoadrenocorticism or Addison's disease and monitoring medical treatment with mitotane or trilostane (ALENZA, 2011; HERRTAGE, 2011).

• Low Dose Dexamethasone Suppression Test: In a normal animal, a low dose of dexamethasone will depress cortisol secretion for more than 8 hours. Dogs with adrenal tumour CAH, cortisol may not be suppressed. In dogs with pituitary-dependent CAH, the cortisol level may rise again in less than 8 hours (KERR, 2003). This low dose test is extremely sensitive and sufficiently specific (LEAL, 2008).

• High Dose Dexamethasone Suppression Test: The aim of this test is to suppress the hypothalamic-pituitary axis and consequently the secretion of ACTH and cortisol for a few hours (PETERSON, 2007). It differentiates pituitary-dependent HAC from adrenal neoplasia (FORD and MAZZAFERRO, 2007).

2.5. Treatment

9

Treatment depends on the aetiology of CAH and may be surgical, clinical or radiotherapy. Regardless of the treatment chosen, they all have side effects, are expensive, require regular monitoring, the co-operation of owners and the knowledge of the veterinary surgeon (MELIÁN, 2012).

2.5.1. Surgical Treatment

When CAH is caused by an adrenal tumour, the recommended treatment is adrenalectomy, which consists of removing the affected gland. Before any procedure it is indicated to perform the metastasis research (AIELLO, 2001).

2.5.2. Clinical Treatment

2.5.2.1. Mitotane

It is a drug with cytotoxic action that causes selective necrosis in the fasciculated and reticular zone of the adrenal (MELIÁN, 2012).

There are two phases in mitotane treatment: an initial induction phase with the administration of 50 mg/kg/day divided into two doses; and a maintenance phase in which the mitotane dosage is reduced to 25 mg/kg/week/ad *eternum* (NELSON, 2006).

2.5.2.2. Ketoconazole

Ketoconazole has low toxicity and reversibly inhibits adrenal steroidogenesis. In general, the dose used is 15 mg/kg BID for the control of CAH (NELSON, 2006).

2.5.2.3. Trilostane

Trilostane is a competitive inhibitor of 3-beta-hydroxysteroid dehydrogenase, an enzyme that catalyses the synthesis of cortisol from cholesterol (FELDMAN, 2011).

A dose of 2 to 6 mg/kg SID is recommended. Subsequently the dose is adjusted based on clinical response (MELIÁN, 2012).

2.5.2.4. Clinical Management of Corticosteroid Remission

The remission in corticoid administration should be gradual, since in cases of abrupt interruption of exogenous glucocorticoid administration, the animal may not be able to respond to the need for endogenous glucocorticoid synthesis, developing Hypoadrenocorticism (LEAL, 2008).

2.5.3. Radiotherapy

Technique reserved for animals with macroadenomas and at risk of developing neurological signs (HÉRIPRET, 2008).

Treatment involves administration of the full radiation dose over a period of 4 to 6 weeks (BIRCHARD & SHERDING, 2003).

Prognosis is based on the relative volume of the tumour and the severity of neurological signs

(NELSON, 2006).

2.6. Complications of Hyperadrenocorticism

Excessive and chronic exposure of the body to glucocorticoids can lead to the development of concomitant clinical changes, the most common of which are:

2.6.1. Systemic Arterial Hypertension

It occurs as a result of sodium retention, activation of the renin-angiotensin system and increased vascular sensitivity to endogenous vasopressors (REUSCH et al., 2010; SMETS et al., 2010). In about 40% of dogs, values tend to remain elevated after initiation of treatment for CAH, due to the presence of atherosclerosis, which induces increased peripheral vascular resistance and reduced sensitivity to vasodilators (SMETS et al., 2010).

Hypertension can induce several systemic complications, such as left ventricular hypertrophy, congestive heart failure, glomerulopathies and pulmonary thromboembolism. Ophthalmic changes resulting from retinal hypertension include intraocular haemorrhage, retinal detachment, secondary glaucoma and blindness (LIEN et al., 2010; REUSCH et al., 2010). Intracranial hypertension can also occur, leading to cerebral oedema and hypertensive encephalopathy (GOY-THOLLOT, 2005).

2.6.2. Diabetes *mellitus*

Dogs with CAH present with hyperglycaemia and hyperinsulinaemia accompanied by marked insulin resistance. Glucocorticoids induce insulin resistance by acting by competitive antagonism with insulin, as well as by reducing the number of insulin receptors in tissues. Affected dogs compensate for this insulin resistance by constant high insulin secretion, which can lead to pancreatic p-cell exhaustion (Herrtage, 2004) and the development of diabetes *mellitus*. CAH should be suspected in dogs treated for Diabetes *mellitus* that do not respond to insulin therapy (MICELI et al., 2012).

2.6.3. Lower Urinary Tract Infection

The potent anti-inflammatory effect of glucocorticoids can suppress the signs of infection, which can occur through a decrease in the body's immune response, the presence of polyuria/polydipsia, poor bladder emptying and the presence of glycosuria (FORRESTER et al., 2003).

These changes, together with the increase in calcium excretion, lead to the appearance of crystalluria, mainly calcium oxalate (ETTINGER & FELDMAN, 2010).

CHAPTER 3

3. GLAUCOMA

According to MILLER (2012), glaucoma is considered one of the major causes of vision loss in dogs. For STROM et al. (2011) glaucoma has an incidence of about 0.5% in dogs.

3.1. Ocular Anatomophysiology

The eye is formed by the ocular bulb, optic nerve and accessory structures (LAUS, 2009).

The bulb can be divided into fibrous, vascular and nervous tunics (LAUS, 2009). Internally, the ocular bulb is divided into aqueous humour, lens and vitreous humour (PIPPI & GONÇALVES, 2009). These structures act in the transmission and refraction of the light ray on the retina and are also responsible for the internal pressure that keeps the globe distended (LAUS, 2009).

The accessory structures (eyelids, conjunctiva, lacrimal apparatus and extraocular muscles) have the function of protecting the bulb (SLATTER, 2005).

The uveal tract is the vascular tunic of the eye. It is formed by the iris, ciliary body and choroid. The iris and ciliary body together are called the anterior uvea (PIPPI & GONÇALVES, 2009). The iris controls the amount of light that enters the eye. Disorders of the iris can affect intraocular pressure (IOP) (SLATTER, 2005).

The ciliary body alters the focusing distance by accommodating the lens and produces the aqueous humour (SLATTER, 2005). This is important in regulating IOP and flows from the posterior chamber to the anterior chamber and the filtration angle (PIPPI & GONÇALVES, 2009). The rate of aqueous humour production is equal to the drainage, keeping it in balance (PERLMANN & RODARTE- ALMEIDA, 2011). Disorders that compromise this balance result in variations in IOP and consequently in glaucoma (SLATTER, 2005).

3.2. Glaucomatous Syndrome

The definition of glaucoma is now broader. Today, in addition to the increase in IOP, manifestations by vascular, cytotoxic and neural pathways are taken into account. The set is called Glaucomatous Syndrome (JUNIOR et al., 2014).

The process results in progressive loss of sensation and function, with retinal ganglion cell death, loss of optic nerve axons, cupping of the optic nerve head, progressive visual field reduction and blindness. Increased IOP is a risk factor for the development of optic neuropathy (MARTINS et al., 2006).

The aqueous humour is responsible for trophic support and removal of metabolites from the cornea and lens. It has a high water concentration and low protein content. It reaches the anterior chamber through the pupil and is drained through the iridocorneal angle and the uveoscleral pathway (unconventional pathway) to reach the blood circulation, maintaining IOP at physiologically acceptable levels (SLATTER, 2005; LAUS, 2009).

In dogs, normal IOP pressure levels range from 12 to 25 mmHg (BORGES et al., 2007). When intraocular pressure is above 25 mmHg, glaucoma is suspected (SLATTER, 2005).
The increase in IOP causes deformity of the cornea, which leads to an increase in the size of the bulb of the

eye (buftalmia) and the sclera due to stretching and thinning of the collagen fibres that compose them (MARTÍN, 2007). Ruptures in the *Descemet*'s membrane also develop with increasing IOP and are observed as linear fissures that can extend across the cornea. Lens dislocation occurs due to disruption of the zonular ligaments (SLATTER, 2005; MARTÍN, 2007) and the passage of fluid, protein, fibrin and blood into the subretinal space, which in the initial phase may have a bubble-like appearance (MAGGIO et al, 2000).

3.3. Classification

Glaucoma can be classified according to the cause (congenital, primary or secondary), the aspect of the drainage angle (open, narrow or closed) and stage of the disease (acute or chronic) (GELATT, 2007).

3.3.1. According to the cause

3.3.1.1. Congenital Glaucoma

Also known as pectinate ligament dysplasia (MARTINS, 2009), it affects dogs before one year of age (STROM et al., 2011).

This disorder is difficult to treat, as many cases end in enucleation due to blindness and therapeutic failure (BERNARDES, 2008).

3.3.1.2. Primary Glaucoma

It occurs due to a hereditary abnormality of the iridocorneal angle, without pre-existing intraocular disorders. There is an elevation of IOP, and in most cases it is bilateral (MILLER, 2012).

Some breeds are predisposed, such as: Basset Hound, Beagle, Cocker Spaniel and Poodle (MARTINS, 2009).

Primary glaucoma is subdivided into primary open-angle glaucoma, whose drainage angle appears normal on gonioscopy, and primary closed-angle glaucoma, whose drainage angle appears narrowed or closed on gonioscopy (MILLER, 2007).

3.3.1.3. Secondary Glaucoma

It is the most common type of glaucoma. The increase in IOP occurs due to pre-existing intraocular disease, which prevents the correct drainage of aqueous humour (MARTINS, 2009). Secondary glaucoma can be uni- or bilateral (MILLER, 2007).

The most frequent causes of secondary glaucoma include uveitis, lens dislocation, hyphema, intraocular neoplasms, and retinal detachment (WILKIE, 2003).

3.3.4. According to the aspect of the drainage angle

Glaucoma will be classified according to the appearance of the iridocorneal angle at gonioscopy, as open, narrow or closed (SLATTER, 2005). Secondary glaucoma will be open-angle, as it is not the primary alteration of the angle that will lead to increased IOP, but a physical barrier to this drainage. Primary glaucoma can be seen with different aspects of drainage angle, the most common being...

3.3.5. According to the stages

The stage of the disease is considered acute when signs are presented for less than two days and chronic with more than five days (MANDELL & HOLT, 2005).

In acute cases, the commonly visualised signs are episcleral hyperemia, corneal oedema, pupillary dilation, pupillary light response and slow to absent threat response, epiphora and blepharospasm (CHIURCIU et al., 2007).

Chronic cases can lead to blindness. The most common clinical changes of chronic glaucoma are retinal and optic nerve degeneration, buftalmia, *descemet's* membrane fractures, absent threat response and photopupillary reflex (BIRCHARD & SHERDING, 2003).

3.4. Clinical Signs

Clinical signs depend on the stage of the disease (ORIA, 2013). In general, clinical signs are occult when the increase in intraocular pressure is mild (levels below 40 mmHg) (MILLER, 2007).

3.4.1. Pain, blepharospasm and behavioural change

Common signs in acute cases. Often the dog rubs the affected eye with its paw, tends to hide and become less sociable (SLATTER, 2005).

3.4.2. Corneal Oedema

Common in both acute and chronic cases of glaucoma. In acute cases, interference with the function of the corneal endothelium by increased IOP and disturbance of the balance between hydration and dehydration in the corneal stroma cause corneal oedema (SLATTER, 2005). In chronic cases, superficial neovascularisation and pigmentation may occur (MARTINS, 2009).

3.4.3. Sclera

In glaucoma, the episcleral veins are engorged and visible (PIPPI and GONÇALVES, 2009). In chronic glaucoma, the sclera distends and the eye increases in volume (buftalmia) (SLATTER, 2005). With the progression of buftalmia, the sclera expands irreversibly, even if IOP is reduced (MARTINS, 2009).

3.4.4. Pupillary diameter

The increase in IOP causes a paralysis of the pupil constrictor muscle, consequently mydriasis occurs. As a result, direct and consensual photopupillary reflexes are impaired (SLATTER, 2005).

3.4.5. Úvea

In persistent IOP elevations, the muscle, iris stroma, body and ciliary processes undergo atrophy. This occurs due to reduced blood supply caused by IOP elevation (SLATTER, 2005).

3.4.6. Lens

Lens dislocation in glaucoma is usually secondary to scleral stretching, uveitis or cataract (SLATTER, 2005). Stretching of the sclera due to increased IOP causes the lenticular zonules to rupture, resulting in lens dislocation (MILLER, 2012).

Increased IOP can also result in cataract (MARTINS, 2009).

3.4.7. Retina and Optic Nerve

In advanced cases, cupping of the optic disc and retinal atrophy may occur, clinically shown by hyper-reflexia of the tapetal area, engorgement of vessels and atrophy of the pigment epithelium of the non-tapetal area (MARTINS, 2009).

3.4.8. Intraocular Pressure

IOP is often increased, but clinical signs should be associated to suspect glaucoma. When glaucoma becomes chronic, the eye bulb becomes buftalmic, i.e. it becomes distended, painful and irreversibly blind. These changes are irreversible even when IOP decreases. Cases of elevated IOP without symptoms may be confused with ocular hypertension (SLATTER, 2005; GELLAT, 1999).

3.5. Diagnosis

Diagnosis can be suggested through clinical and ophthalmic examination, associated with history, race, and age (MILLER, 2012).

IOP can be altered by changes in osmotic and blood pressures, intraocular inflammation, method of containment, tonometrist and the tonometer used (SLATTER, 2005; COLITZ, 2007).

The most routine tests for the diagnosis of glaucoma include ophthalmoscopy, gonioscopy and applanation tonometry. Ultrasonography and electroretinography complement the above tests (MARTINS, 2009).

3.5.1. Ophthalmoscopy

Direct and indirect ophthalmoscopy are recommended for glaucomatous patients and can be used to examine the optic nerve and retina (SLATTER, 2005). However, the opacity of transparent media may prevent performance (TALIERI et al., 2006). On ophthalmoscopy, cupping of the optic disc can be seen, with grey to whitish colouration; tapetal hyperreflexia with attenuation of retinal vessels; retinal detachment and optic atrophy (CHIURCIU et al., 2007).

3.5.2. Gonioscopy

It assesses the condition of the anterior chamber drainage angle and contributes to the selection of an appropriate therapeutic approach. It is usually performed with a Koeppe lens, which should be gently positioned on the cornea after instillation of anaesthetic eye drops and methylcellulose solution. Allied to the aid of a portable biomicroscope or direct ophthalmoscope, the condition and characteristics of the iridocorneal angle can be visualised (MARTINS, 2009).

3.5.3. Tonometry

Technique that determines intraocular pressure. Used for diagnosis and for monitoring cases (MARTINS, 2009).

Tonometry is classified according to the diagnostic instrument used as indentation, flattening and rebound (MARTINS, 2009; PEREIRA, 2010).

3.5.3.1. Indentation Tonometry

The *Schiotz* indentation instrument is low cost and easy to manipulate in veterinary medicine (MARTINS, 2009).

In this technique, a standardised force of the metal rod is applied to the anaesthetised cornea. The distance that the rod indents the cornea is related to the intraocular pressure (SLATTER, 2005).

3.5.3.2. Flattening Tonometry

Applanation tonometry is the most recommended technique in veterinary medicine (BORGES et al., 2007). The Tono-Pen® XL (Reichert) is the most widespread device. After reading, the result, in mm Hg, is presented on the liquid crystal display (MARTINS, 2009). Its small base makes it possible to obtain a reading just by contacting a small area of the cornea (COLITZ, 2007). It is suitable for all types of patients.

3.5.3.3. Rebound Tonometry

This technique measures IOP non-invasively. It is calibrated according to the animal species. Six contacts with the cornea are required for the mean IOP to be determined, without the need for anaesthetic eye drops. It measures pressures from 1 - 99 mmHg (PEREIRA, 2010).

Rebound tonometry, in animal studies, has a tendency to underestimate IOP. It can also be influenced by corneal properties such as corneal hysteresis and corneal resistance factor (PEREIRA, 2010).

3.5.4. Ocular ultrasound

Ultrasonography is a non-invasive and complementary examination, assisting in determining the size of ocular structures and in the diagnosis of ocular size abnormalities (BRANDÃO et al., 2007).

In eyes with opacification of transparent media, ultrasound imaging allows observation of optic disc cupping (MARTINS, 2009).

3.5.5. Electroretinography

It assesses the response of retinal cells to a light stimulus. In glaucomatous patients, there is a decreased response to light stimuli, since the ganglion cells are affected (MARTINS, 2009).

3.6. Treatment

The choice of the best treatment depends on the cause and stage of glaucoma (SLATTER 2005). Clinical treatment aims to decrease aqueous humour production or increase its drainage to prevent optic nerve damage, preserve visual function and decrease pain sensitivity (BORGES et al., 2007).

Surgical treatment aims to develop an alternative route for aqueous humour drainage (MARTINS, 2009).

3.6.1. Surgical Treatment

Glaucoma can often become refractory to drug therapy over the course of treatment (ORIA, 2013). The aim is to relieve ocular pain and discomfort (CHIURCIU et al., 2007).

3.6.1.1. Increased drainage of aqueous humour

Surgical procedures that aim to increase aqueous humour drainage are known as filtering operations. These often result in failure as a scar, which forms within a short time, plugs the constructed drainage space (KASECKER & WOUK, 2003).

Scleral trephination associated with peripheral iridectomy allows the construction of a drainage fistula of adequate size to maintain filtration, in addition to being an easy technique to perform (KASECKER & WOUK, 2003).

Anterior chamber gonioimplants (*shunts*) are used to increase aqueous humour drainage. They are devices that create an alternative route for aqueous humour drainage (MARTINS, 2009).

3.6.1.2. Cyclocryothermia

It consists of the application of liquid nitrogen or nitrous oxide to the ciliary body, with the aim of producing necrosis of the ciliary body by freezing (MARTÍN, 2007).

Postoperative complications include chemosis, pain, blepharospasm, uveitis, choroidal effusion, retinal detachment and *phthisis bulbi* (MARTINS, 2009).

3.6.1.3. Laser Therapy

The laser makes it possible to treat an eye with intermittent increases in pressure, but which remains visual. This technique has a reduced reaction of the ocular tissues, with less postoperative swelling and irritation (SLATTER, 2005).

3.6.1.4. Intrascleral prosthesis

The prosthesis is intended to improve aesthetics, since the loss of the ocular bulb is disfiguring (RAHAL et al., 2000).

Evisceration is indicated in cases of buftalmia, permanent blindness, after corneal or scleral laceration, in hyphema resulting from retinal dislocation or in chronic painful uveitis (RAHAL et al., 2000).

The procedure consists of applying a prosthesis inside the bulb of the eye, after evisceration of its contents. The materials generally used are silicone, double-pleated tricalcium phosphate cement or polymethylmethacrylate and acrylic resin (MARTINS, 2009).

3.6.1.5. Chemical Ablation of the Ciliary Body

The technique aims to cause pharmacological destruction, by toxic necrosis of the ciliary body, through intravitreal injection of gentamicin sulphate and dexamethasone (MARTINS, 2009). It is contraindicated in cases of neoplasia or ocular inflammation (BROOKS, 2008).

This procedure allows the maintenance of the bulb of the eye by reducing its size to near normal, prevents ocular pain and presents a good aesthetic result (CHIURCIU et al., 2007).

3.6.2. Clinical Treatment

3.6.2.1. Osmotic Diuretics

Osmotic agents (mannitol and glycerol) are used in acute and emergency cases (MARTINS, 2009).

Osmotic diuretics cross the blood-aqueous and haematoretinal barriers and, by osmotic gradient, remove water, causing a decrease in IOP; a decrease in vitreous volume and clearance of corneal oedema (ANDRADE, 2008).

Mannitol and glycerol should be used immediately in cases where IOP values remain between 50 and 60 mmHg for more than 24 to 48 hours, which may result in irreversible vision loss (SLATTER, 2005).

3.6.2.2. Cholinergic agents

These drugs increase the drainage angle and consequently facilitate the drainage of aqueous humour (ANDRADE, 2008).

Pilocarpine is indicated as an adjuvant in the control of primary glaucoma in dogs (MARTINS, 2009), as it promotes ciliary muscle contraction (ANDRADE, 2008).

However, it is contraindicated in secondary glaucoma as its myopathic effect predisposes to breakdown of the blood-air barrier, posterior synechia and pupillary occlusion, exacerbating the pain and symptoms of uveitis (BROOKS, 2008).

Intracameral application of carbacol 0.01% prevents postoperative intraocular hypertension caused by phacoemulsification (MARTINS, 2009).

3.6.2.3. Adrenergic agents

Adrenaline reduces aqueous humour production and increases outflow (Moore, 2003).

Brimonidine tartrate significantly lowers IOP, causes miosis and reduces heart rate (MARTINS, 2009).

3.6.2.4. Antiadrenergic agents

P-adrenergic blockers cause a decrease in IOP (MARTINS, 2009).

Timolol is used to treat primary and secondary glaucoma (MOORE, 2003), but is contraindicated in patients with heart problems because it causes a decrease in heart rate in dogs and cats (MARTINS, 2009).

3.6.2.5. Carbonic Anhydrase Inhibitors (CAI)

ACEIs reduce IOP by blocking the enzyme carbonic anhydrase, which is present in the ciliary body and is responsible for the active production of aqueous humour (BROOKS, 2008). These drugs also inhibit carbonic anhydrase in the renal tubular epithelium, causing diuresis (SLATTER, 2005).

For additional hypotensive effects, in cases of glaucoma, CAIs are administered in combination with other agents (Moore, 2003).

3.6.2.6. Prostaglandin analogues

Prostaglandin analogues are preferably used in cases of primary glaucoma, as they increase the drainage of aqueous humour through the uveoscleral route. They have greater ocular hypotensive effects (MARTINS, 2009).

It is contraindicated in patients with glaucoma secondary to uveitis, since the aqueous humour in these conditions is already rich in prostaglandins and in cases of anterior lens dislocation, as they are highly myotic and may trigger acute pupillary block and vitreous incarceration (WILLIS, 2004).

CHAPTER 4

4. CASE REPORT: GLAUCOMA INDUCED BY IATROGENIC HYPERADRENOCORTICISM

4.4. History and anamnesis

A 12-year-old male Shih Tzu weighing 5kg was treated at the Veterinary Hospital of the Federal University of Goiás, Jataí Region.

The owner reported conjunctival hyperaemia in the left eye, emesis, apathy, bloody urine, dermatological lesions such as: intense pruritus, crusted lesions in the abdominal region, perilabial and on the back.

The dog had already undergone dermatological care three years ago, and since then the owner has been giving the animal glucocorticoids every 48 hours.

4.5. Physical Examination

On physical assessment, the patient's general condition was normal. He had a temperature of 38.3° Celsius, a heart rate of 88 beats per minute and tachypnoea.

Dermatological assessment showed hair thinning, yellowish crusted lesions on the skin (abdominal, perilabial and dorsal), presence of ectoparasites, erythema and thinning.

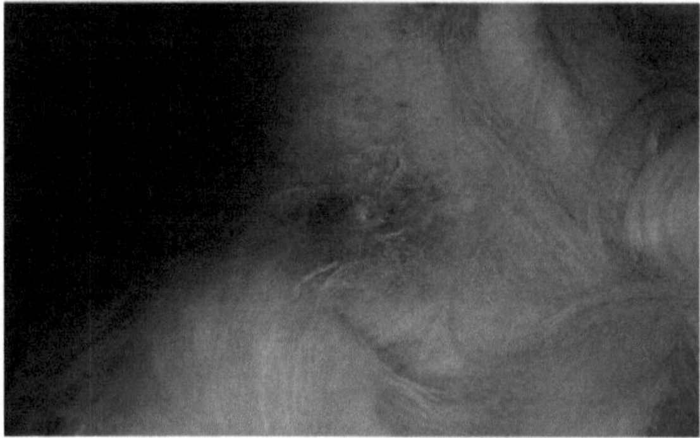

FIGURA 1:   Abdominal lesion with presence of yellowish crusts. Note the intensity of the erythema. Source: Personal archive - 2015.

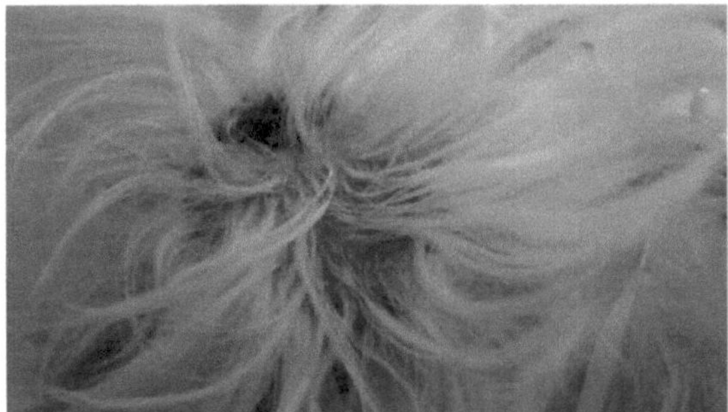

FIGURA 2:   Hyperemic perilabial lesion. Source: Personal archive - 2015.

4.6. Ophthalmological examination

Observation of the size of the eyeballs revealed buftalmia of the left eye (Figure 3).

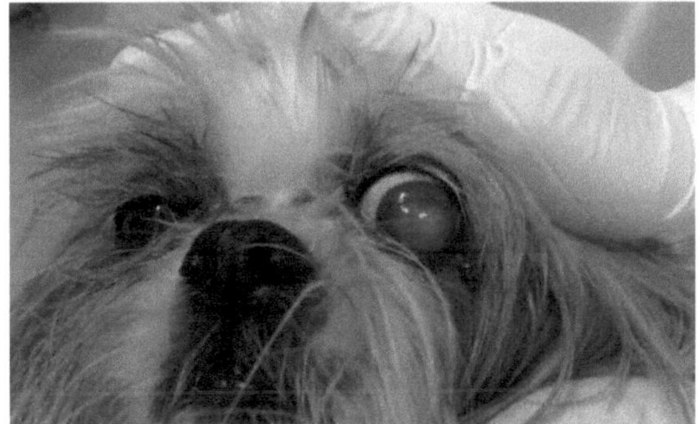

FIGURE 3: Patient showing buftalmia and marked corneal oedema in the left eye. Source: Personal Archive - 2015.

For the ophthalmological examination, a slit-lamp biomicroscope (SL-14 Kowa, Japan), applanation tonometry (Tonopen XL, Mentor), direct (Heine, Germany) and indirect ophthalmoscopy (IO-H, Neitz), sodium fluorescein strips (Fluorescein Strips, Ophthalmos, SP, Brazil) and Koeppe lens for gonioscopy (Koeppe medium diagnostic lens 18 mm - Ocular) were used.

Direct and indirect photopupillary reflexes were absent in the right eye. It was not possible to check these reflexes in the left eye due to marked corneal opacity, preventing observation of pupillary diameter. Threat response was absent in both eyes.

In the left eye (Figure 4), there was marked corneal opacity with diffuse oedema throughout the cornea and engorgement of the episcleral vessels. It was not possible to visualise the anterior chamber by biomicroscopy and the posterior ocular segment by direct or indirect ophthalmoscopy, due to the intense opacity throughout the cornea.

Mydriasis and anterior chamber enlargement were observed in the right eye on biomicroscopy. Indirect ophthalmoscopy showed some retinal haemorrhage.

Intraocular pressure in the right eye was 46 mmHg and in the right eye 84 mmHg, measured after instillation of 0.5% proximetacaine eye drops (Anestalcon®). The fluorescein dye test was negative in both eyes.

Gonioscopy was possible only in the right eye, performed after new instillation of 0.5% proximetacaine eye drops and three drops of sterile ophthalmic solution of hypromellose (Filmcel®). A Koeppe lens was placed on the cornea and observation of the iridocorneal angle was made with biomiscroscopy, showing no abnormality.

4.7. Additional examinations

Complete blood count with platelet count and haematozoa count, serum biochemistry (urea, creatinine, ALT and FA), urinalysis, IOP measurement by tonometry, abdominal and ocular ultrasound, skin scraping, culture and antibiogram were performed, as well as hormonal tests: thyroid stimulating hormone (TSH), cortisol, triglycerides, cholesterol, total and free thyroxine (total T4 and free T4).

4.7.1. Full Blood Count

Erythrogram values were within the reference range for the species. The leucogram showed intense leucocytosis, neutrophilia with regenerative left shift, absolute eosinophilia and absolute lymphopenia. Platelet count within normal range and no presence of haematozoa.

4.7.2. Serum Biochemistry

Serum biochemistry showed altered values for ALT 300 U/L (reference 10 to 80 U/L) and FA 2927 U/L (reference 20 to 150 U/L). Urea and creatinine values were within normal parameters.

4.7.3. Urinalysis

Changes in urinalysis consist of alkaline pH, proteinuria, bilirubinuria, haematuria, pyuria, with presence of amorphous phosphate crystals and struvite.

4.7.4. Abdominal and ocular ultrasonography

For the ultrasound evaluation, Samsung Medison equipment was used, model Sonoace 3, with linear, multi-frequency transducer (5 to 12 MHz), selected for better resolution (12 MHz).

Ultrasonography assessed the liver, gallbladder, spleen, gastrointestinal system, adrenals, kidneys, prostate and bladder. Only the gallbladder, adrenals and bladder were outside the normal range. The gallbladder was greatly enlarged, bilateral adrenal hypoplasia and cystitis were found.

On ocular ultrasound, the left side had preserved contours, with axial length measuring 2.32 cm, enlarged anterior chamber (0.60 cm), normal lens (0.66 cm), enlarged vitreous chamber (1.1 cm), optic nerve region and retro bulbar space with no noteworthy sonographic changes. Highly reflective punctate echoes in the vitreous chamber, suspended and retinal detachment were noted (Figure 5).

On the right side, the eye showed preserved contours, normal axial length (2.28 cm), normal anterior chamber (0.28 cm), decreased lens (0.6 cm), increased vitreous chamber (1.16 cm). There was presence of membranous echoes in vitreous chamber in addition to retinal detachment. Both eyes were suggestive of buftalmia.

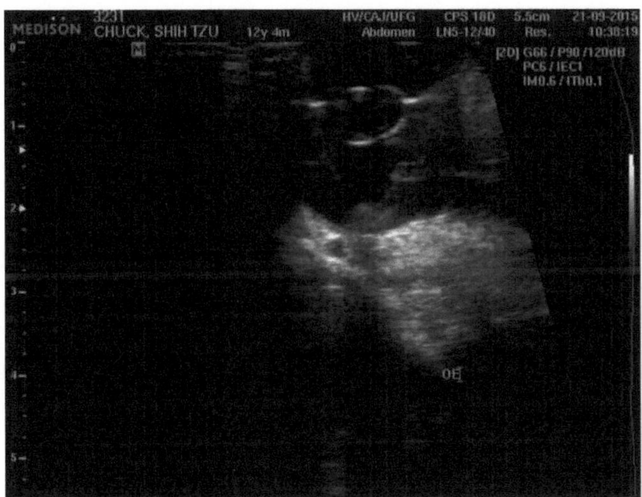

FIGURE 4: Complete detached retinal membranes from the optic disc for *ora serrata*. Source: Personal archive - 2015.

4.7.5. Dermatological assessments

Nothing was visualised in the scraping. In the skin culture and antibiogram, *Escherichia coli* was isolated.

4.7.6. Endocrine tests

TSH, free T4 and cortisol were normal, total T4 was below normal and cholesterol and triglycerides were increased compared to the reference values for the species.

4.8. Treatment

In view of the clinical picture that the patient presented, Cosopt (1 drop in each eye, BID), Ranitidine (2 mg/Kg, VO, TID), Metoclopramide (0.2 mg/Kg, VO, BID), Hydroxyzine (2.2 mg/Kg, VO, TID), Ursacol (100 mg/Kg, VO, SID), SAME (20 mg/Kg, SID, VO), Hepvet (half tablet, VO, SID), Cortavance Topical on skin lesions, Chlorhexidine Shampoo (two baths per week for 4 weeks) and Chlorhexidine 0.5% topical on lesions.

Glucocorticoid withdrawal occurred gradually and with weekly follow-ups.

With the results of the culture and antibiogram, the antibiotic of choice was Norfloxacin (15 mg/kg, VO, BID).

CHAPTER 5

5. DISCUSSION

CAH is one of the most common endocrine diseases in dogs. It usually affects middle-aged to elderly animals. The most predisposed breeds are Poodles, the breeds of Terriers, Beagles, Dachshund and German Shepherd. However, it can affect any breed (LOPES, 2011). In this case report, the animal was 12 years old and was of the Shih Tzu breed.

Most dogs with this syndrome show signs that progress slowly and are not alarming to owners (OLIVEIRA, 2004). This is confirmed by the proposed study, since three years passed before the owner of the animal took him to a new consultation with an ophthalmological focus.

In this study, some common skin lesions of canine CAH were observed, such as: dull coat, easily shaved hair, thinner skin, pruritus and presence of bacterial pyoderma. This is due to the immunosuppressive effect of excess cortisol, corroborating the studies by SCARAMPELLA, 2011 and OLIVEIRA, 2012.

From the first consultation, the dog attended presented tachypnoea. According to ALENZA (2011), in cases of CAH, the dog has short breaths with a rapid rest period. This is due to increased fat deposition on the thorax, loss of musculature and weakness of the muscles involved in breathing.

Urinary tract infections are common in dogs with CAH. Decreased resistance to infections may result from glucocorticoid-induced inhibition (REIS, 2009). *Escherichia coli* is the most frequently isolated bacterium in urinary tract infections secondary to CAH (LEAL, 2008). The affected dog had recurrent cystitis and was difficult to treat, as it was already resistant to most antibiotics.

According to Nichols (1994), about 5% to 10% of dogs with CAH have urinary calculi containing calcium. Calcium oxalate and calcium phosphate uroliths are more commonly found in cases of CAH, as corticoids increase urinary calcium excretion. However, the presence of urinary infection and triple phosphate crystals in the sediment does not rule out the occurrence of struvite uroliths, which precipitate at alkaline pH, which occurs in cystitis (FELDMAN, 1997).

On urinalysis, consistent changes were already present. The urine was alkaline, there was proteinuria, bilirubinuria, haematuria, pyuria, with the presence of amorphous phosphate and struvite crystals and other changes. A treatment was started immediately to prevent the formation of uroliths, which are common in this disease. As for proteinuria, it can be caused by glomerulopathies, systemic hypertension, or by lower urinary tract infection (ALENZA, 2011).

The most frequent alteration found in the haemogram of a dog with CAH is the "stress leucogram", i.e. neutrophilia, monocytosis, lymphopenia and eosinopenia, caused by excessive cortisol production (ETTINGER & FELDMAN, 2010), but in the present case the eosinophils were increased, possibly due to the allergic condition presented by the patient.

The cortisol value was within the reference for the species, however, the dosage of the basal level of cortisol has no definitive diagnostic value because it is secreted sporadically during the day (FELDMAN, 2004).

Chemical abnormalities may appear through serum as increased activity of FA, ALT and hypercholesterolaemia (SILVA, 2013). These data are in accordance with what is found in the examinations carried out periodically in the animal.

Increased ALT occurs due to hepatocellular necrosis, glycogen accumulation or interference with hepatic blood flow (ALENZA, 2011). 15. 15 Increased FA is the most common laboratory alteration in canine CAH. The steroid-dependent alkaline phosphatase isoenzyme (SFAI) is a major contributor to the increase in FA concentration as it is induced by glucocorticoids at the level of the hepatocyte bile canaliculi membrane (KOOISTRA & GALAC, 2010). Hypercholesterolaemia and hypertriglycaemia occur due to glucocorticoid stimulation of lipolysis (ALENZA, 2011).

On ultrasound, adrenal hypoplasia was noted, which contrasts with the data studied by APTEKMANN (2003) who found an increase in the adrenals. Regarding the findings of ocular ultrasound, according to CARVALHO (2014), the axial length can vary from 1.7 cm to 2.3 cm; the anterior chamber from 0.28 cm to 0.54 cm; the lens from 0.65 cm to 0.81 cm and the vitreous chamber: 0.8 cm to 1.0 cm, which goes according to the animal's presentation.

Hypertension is a relatively common finding in dogs with CAH. One of the main indications for assessing blood pressure in a patient is the observation of clinical changes with hypertensive ocular (hypertensive retinopathy), renal, cardiovascular and neurological damage (TEBALDI, 2011).

Healthy dogs have a systolic, diastolic and mean blood pressure of 150, 90, 105 mmHg, respectively. Dogs affected by Cushing's syndrome have an average blood pressure of 162, 116, 135 mmHg, respectively. The dog had a systemic blood pressure of 160 mmHg (MATTOS, 2012).

The development of hypertension may have multiple factors, such as: cortisol activity that can increase renal hydrosodic retention and consequently volemia; increased activity of the renin angiotensin system; potentiation of the action of catecholamines by increased sensitivity of the myocardium and vascular walls and a reduction in vasodilator prostaglandins (LEAL, 2008).

Hypertension tends to resolve with successful treatment of Cushing's syndrome, but secondary changes can occur. Ophthalmological complications are recurrent and can lead to glaucoma and blindness due to retinal haemorrhage or detachment (LEAL, 2008). Recovery of vision following retinal detachment or pronounced hyphema is rare (JEPSON, 2011).

The ophthalmic signs presented by this animal are common in patients with CAH and secondary hypertension. The ocular changes observed occur mainly in chronic cases gradually, in which excessive increases in blood pressure affect the retinal self-regulation mechanism, which is not able to contain hypertension and ends up presenting important changes (QUEIROZ et al., 2015).

The initial sign of hypertensive retinopathy is visual impairment, followed by haemorrhage and retinal detachment. Other changes are also observed, such as narrowing of the retinal arterioles, ischaemic spots in the retina, tortuosity of the retinal arterioles, signs of perivasculitis, papilledema, retinal oedema, retinal microaneurysms, arteriovenous crossing and tapetal hyperreflexia (QUEIROZ et al., 2015).

Glaucoma decreased with treatment, but did not return to normal values for the species (10 and 25 mmHg). The increase in IOP favours engorgement of episcleral vessels and conjunctival hyperemia (MARTINS et al., 2006). The observed buftalmia is due to the stretching and thinning of the collagen fibres that compose them, which causes deformity of the cornea and sclera (MARTÍN, 2007). Corneal oedema occurs due to the rapid elevation of IOP, which alters the function of the corneal endothelium, in addition to the acquired opacification of the cornea (MARTINS et al., 2006).

Unresponsive pupillary dilation or mydriasis, due to rapid IOP elevation, causes impaired blood and nerve supply to the central region of the iris. Retinal ganglion cell dysfunction also contributes to mydriasis (MARTINS et al., 2006).

The retina normally attaches to the optic nerve posteriorly and the *ora serrata* anteriorly. With detachment, the layers of the retina remain attached to these points but may be separated from the choroid by fluid between them. Causes of retinal detachment include hypermature cataract, trauma, inflammation, tumours or systemic hypertension (PENNINCK & ANJOU, 2011).

CHAPTER 6

6. CONCLUSIONS

CAH is a common endocrinopathy in routine Veterinary Medicine that presents a variety of clinical signs and its diagnosis is made through history, clinical signs, physical examination and complementary tests that will help to conclude the diagnosis and consequently an appropriate treatment.

Glaucoma affects several eye structures, causing lesions that are most often associated with increased intraocular pressure. Owners rarely notice any eye changes in their pet, which makes successful treatment difficult.

Lack of clarification on the part of the owner leads to damage to the animal. It is important to emphasise that all treatment depends, to a large extent, on the owner's contribution and incorrect management compromises the treatment and even more the animal's health.

CHAPTER 7

BIBLIOGRAPHICAL REFERENCES

ABREU, D. R. G. **Cutaneous manifestations associated with endocrinopathies in dogs**. Vila Real, 2012, 84f. Dissertation (Integrated Master in Veterinary Medicine) - Veterinary Sciences, University of Trás-Os-Montes and Alto Douro.

AIELLO, S. E. **Merck Manual of Veterinary Medicine**. 8 ed. São Paulo: Roca, 2001. 1860 p.

ALENZA, D. P. Hyperadrenocorticism: Are we over-diagnosing it? **Proceedings of the Southern European Conference & Congreso Nacional AVEPA**. Barcelona, 2011.

ANDRADE, S. F. **Manual of Veterinary Therapeutics**. São Paulo: Roca, 2008. 936 p.

APTEKMANN, K. P.; PEIXOTO, A. S.; ALTWEGG, O.; VICENTE, P. C.; SCHWARTZ, D. S. Clinical-epidemiological characteristics of hyperadrenocorticism in the region of Botucatu - SP. **Braz. J. vet. Res. animo Sci**, São Paulo, v. 40, supplement, p. 192 - 193. 2003.

BERNARDES, J. R. **Treatment of Canine Glaucoma**. 2008. 76f. Dissertation (Master), Technical University of Lisbon.

BIRCHARD, S. J.; SHERDING, R. G. **Saunders Manual - Small Animal Clinic**. 2ª ed. São Paulo: Roca, 2003. 2072 p.

BORGES, A. G.; BRANDÃO, C. V. S.; RANZANI, J. J. T.; ADALBERTO, J. C. Effects of timolol maleate 0.5% dorzolamide hydrochloride 2%, and the association of both on intraocular pressure. **Arquivo Brasileiro de Medicina Veterinária e Zootecnia**, Belo Horizonte, v. 59, n. 3, p. 660 - 664. 2007.

BRANDÃO, C.V.S.; CHIURCIU, J. L. V.; RANZANI, J. J. T.; MAMPRIM, M. J.; ZANINI, M.; CROCCI, J. A. Tonometry, pachymetry and ocular axial length in glaucomatous dogs submitted to intravitreal uveal ablation. **Arquivo Brasileiro de Medicina Veterinária e Zootecnia**, Belo Horizonte, v. 59, n. 4, p. 914 - 919. 2007.

BROOKS, D. E. Glaucoma. In: HERRERA, D. H. **Clinical Ophthalmology in Companion Animals**. São Paulo: MEDVET, 2008. p.195 - 203.

CARVALHO, C. F. **Ultrasonography in Small Animals**. 2. ed. São Paulo: Roca, 2014, 468p.

CARVALHO, L. A. **Hyperadrenocorticism (Cushing's Syndrome)**. Portal Educação [online]. Available at: http://www.portaleducacao.com.br/veterinaria/artigos/3569/hiperadrenocorticismo-	sindrome-de-mes. January 2008. Html. [Captured on 12 Dec. 2015].

CHIURCIU, J. L. V. BRANDÃO, C. V. S.; RANZANI, J. J. T.; CREMONINI, D. N.; CROCCI, J. A. Clinical evaluation of intravitreal uveal ablation with gentamicin in dogs with chronic glaucoma.

Arquivo Brasileiro de Medicina Veterinária e Zootecnia, Belo Horizonte, v. 59, n. 2, p. 345 - 349. 2007.

COLITZ, C. M. H. Glaucoma: What Can I Do Before I Send It? **North American Veterinary Conference**.

Gainsville, p. 815 - 817. 2007.

ETTINGER, S. J.; FELDMAN, E. C. Hyperadrenocorticism. In: **Texbook of Veterinary Internal Medicine**. Philadelphia: W. B. Saunders, 2010. p. 1460 - 1487.

FELDMAN, E. C. Hyperadrenocorticism. In: ETTINGER, S. J.; FELDMAN, E. C. **Treatise on veterinary internal medicine**. São Paulo: Manole, 1997. p. 2123.

FELDMAN, E. C. Hyperadrenocorticism. In: ETTINGER, S. J.; FELDMAN, E. C. **Treatise on veterinary internal medicine - Diseases of the dog and cat** (Ed.). São Paulo: Guanabara Koogan, 2004. p. 2236.

FELDMAN, E. C. Evaluation of twice-daily lower-dose trilostane treatment administered orally in dogs with naturally occurring hyperadrenocorticism. **J Am Vet Med Assoc**, Illinois, v. 238, p. 1441 - 1451. 2011.

FELDMAN, E. C. Diagnosis of Hyperadrenocorticism (Cushing's Syndrome) in dogs. Which tests are best? In: **VII Congress of the Montenegro Veterinary Hospital**. Santa Maria da Feira, Portugal. 2012.

FORD, R. B.; MAZZAFERRO, E. M. **Manual of Veterinary Procedures and Emergency Treatment, according to Kirk and Bestner**. São Paulo: Roca, 2007. 768 p.

FORRESTER, S. D.; MARTINEZ, N. I.; PANCIERA, D. L.; MOON, M. L.; PICKETT, C. R.; WARD, D. L. Absence of urinary tract infection in dogs with experimentally induced hyperadrenocorticism. **Res Vet Sci**, Rome, v. 74, n. 2, p. 179 - 182. 2003.

GELATT, K. N. Veterinary Ophthalmology.3. ed. Philadelphia: Lippincott Williams & Wilkins, 1999, 760p.

GELLAT, K. N. **Veterinary ophthalmology**. Philadelphia: Oxford Blackwell Publishing Ltd, 2007. 1696 p.

GILOR, C.; GRAVES, T. K. Interpretation of laboratory tests for canine Cushing's syndrome. **Top Companion Anim Med,** Amsterdam, n. 26, v. 2, p. 98 - 108. 2011.

GOY-THOLLOT, I.oy-Thollot I. (2005) **Consequences hemodynamiques et electrolytiques de 1'agression, de l'hypercorticisme hypophysaire et du vieillissement chez le chien - role de la secretion cortico-surrenalienne**, 2005. Thesis (PhD) - Ecole Nationale Veterinaire de Lyon, France. 2005.

HÉRIPRET, D. Cuhsing Syndrome. In: GUAGUÉRE, E.; PRÉLAUD, P.; CRAIG, M. (Eds.). **A Practical Guide to Canine Dermatology**. Merial: Kaliantis, 2008. p. 337-347.

HERRTAGE, M. E. Canine Hyperadrenocorticism. In: MOONEY, C. T.; PETERSON, M. E. (Eds.). **BSAVA Manual of Canine and Feline Endocrinology**. Gloucester: BSAVA, 2004. p. 150-171.

HERRTAGE, M. E. Diagnosing canine hyperadrenocorticism. In: **Proceedings of the 36th world small animal veterinary congress, WSAVA**. Korea, 2011.

JEPSON R. E. Feline systemic hypertension: Classification and pathogenesis. **J Feline Med Surg**, London, v. 13, n. 1, p. 25 - 34. 2011.

JUNIOR, A. Z.; ZACARIAS, F. G. S.; CARDOSO, M. J.. L.; BRACARENSE, A. P. F. R. L. Canine glaucoma and Helicobacter spp. infection: a possible correlation. **Semina: Ciências Agrárias**, Londrina, v. 35, n. 4, p. 1973 - 1984. 2014.

KASECKER, G. G.; WOUK, A. F. de F. Filtering Surgical Treatment of Glaucoma Associated with Topical Use of Salicylic Acid in Dogs. **Revista Acadêmica: Ciências Agrárias e Ambientais,** Curitiba, v. 1, n. 4, p. 67-74. 2003.

KERR, M. G. **Laboratory tests in veterinary medicine: clinical biochemistry and haematology**. São Paulo: Roca, 2003.433 p.

KOOISTRA, H. S.; GALAC, S. Recent advances in the diagnosis of Cushings syndrome in dogs. **Vet Clin North Am Small Anim Pract,** Amsterdam, v. 40, n. 2, p. 259 - 267. 2010.

LEAL, R. O. **Approach to the Diagnosis of Canine Hyperadrenocorticism: Importance of Functional Tests**. Lisbon, 2008, 181f. Dissertation (Integrated Master in Veterinary Medicine) - Faculty of Veterinary Medicine, Technical University of Lisbon.

LAUS, J. L. **Clinical and surgical ophthalmology in dogs and cats**. São Paulo: Roca, 2009. 248 p.

LIEN, Y.; HSIANG, T.; HUANG, H. Associations among systemic blood pressure, microalbuminuria and albuminuria in dogs affected with pituitary- and adrenal- dependent hyperadrenocorticism. **Acta veterinaria scandinava**, Copenhagen, p. 52 - 61. 2010.

LIMA, V. G. **Laboratory changes caused by hyperadrenocorticism in dogs and cats: a review**. Rio de Janeiro, 2008, 31f. Post-graduation course conclusion work (Veterinary clinical pathology course) - Instituto Qualittas, Universidade Castelo Branco.

LOPES, K. G. P. A. **Hyperadrenocorticism in dogs**. Goiânia, 2011, 25f. Postgraduate course conclusion work - Qualittas Institute, Castelo Branco University.

MAGGIO, F.; DEFRANCESCO, T. C.; ATKINS, C. E. Ocular lesions associated with systemic hypertension in cats: 69 cases (1985-1998). **Journal of Veterinary Medicine Association**, New York, v. 217, n. 5, p. 695 - 702. 2000.

MANDELL, D. C; HOLT, E. Ophthalmic Emergencies. **Veterinary Clinics of North America: Small Animal Practice,** Missouri, v. 35, p. 455 - 480. 2005.

MARTÍN, J. E. Ophthalmological Emergencies. **Atlas de Oftalmología Clinica Del Perro y Del Gato.** Zaragoza: Servet, 2007. 344 p.

MARTINS, B. C.; VICENTI, F. A. M.; LAUS, J. L. Glaucomatous syndrome in dogs - part 1. **Ciência Rural**, Santa Maria, v. 36, n. 6, p. 1952 - 1958, 2006.

MARTINS, B. C. Glaucoma. In: LAUS, J. L. (Ed.). **Clinical and Surgical Ophthalmology in Dogs and Cats.** São Paulo: Roca, 2009. p.151-167.

MASCHIETTO, L. A. **Sex steroid profile in dogs with hyperadrenocorticism- diagnostic aspect and clinical correlations**. São Paulo, 2007, 89f. Dissertation (Master in Veterinary Clinic) - Faculty of Veterinary Medicine and Zootechny, University of São Paulo.

MATTOS, A. H. A. F. **Evaluation of blood pressure by vascular doppler measurement and retinography of hypertensive dogs**. Brasília, 2012, 86f. Dissertation (Master in Animal Health) - Faculty of Agronomy and

Veterinary Medicine, University of Brasilia.

MELIÁN, C. **Tratamiento del Hiperadrenocorticism (Síndrome de Cushing).** Lisbon, 2012, 10f. Communication (Post-Graduation in Companion Animal Medicine), Technical University of Lisbon.

MICELI, D. D.; GALLELLI, M. F.; BLATTER, M. F.; MARTIARENA, B.; BRANAS, M. M.; ORTEMBERG, L. R. Low dose of insulin detemir controls glycaemia, insulinemia and prevents diabetes mellitus progression in the dog with pituitary-dependent hyperadrenocorticism. **Res Vet Sci,** Amsterdam, v. 93, n. 1, p. 114-120. 2012.

MILLER, P. E. **Manual of Small Animal Surgery**. São Paulo: Manole, 2007. 2896 p.

MOORE, C. P. **Pharmacology and Therapeutics in Veterinary.** Rio de Janeiro: GUANABARA KOOGAN, 2003. 1048 p.

NELSON, R. W. Disorders of the adrenal gland. In: NELSON, R. W.; COUTO, C. G. (Ed.). **Small animal internal medicine**. Rio de Janeiro: Elseirer Ltda, 2006. p. 824 - 862.

NELSON, R. W.; COUTO, C. G. **Manual of Small Animal Internal Medicine**. 2. ed. São Paulo: Mosby, 2006. 1128 p.

NELSON, R.; COUTO, C. **Small Animal Internal Medicine**, 4 ed. St. Louis: Mosby, 2009. p. 778 - 798.

NICHOLS, R.; PETERSON, M. E.; MULLER, H. S. Adrenal glands. In: BIRCHARD, S. S.; SHERDING, R. G. **Small animal clinic**. Roca: São Paulo, 1998. p. 272 - 281.

OLIVEIRA, S. T. **Disorders of adrenal hormones in dogs**. Rio Grande do Sul, 2004, 18f. Seminar of the Post-graduation course - Veterinary Sciences Sector, Federal University of Rio Grande do Sul.

OLIVEIRA, A. M. Cutaneous manifestations of endocrine diseases. In: **VII Congress of the Montenegro Veterinary Hospital**. Santa Maria da Feira, Portugal. 2012.

ORIÁ, A. P.; GOMES JUNIOR, D. C.; SOUZA, M. R.; COSTA NETO, J. M.; ESTRELA-LIMA, A.; DÓREA NETO, F. A. Secondary glaucoma in dogs and cats. **Medicina Veterinária**, Recife, v. 7, n. 3, p. 13 - 22. 2013.

PENNINCK, D.; ANJOU, M. A. **Atlas of Small Animal Ultrasonography**. 1. ed. Rio de Janeiro: Guanabara Koogan, 2011, 513p.

PEREIRA, F. Q. **Comparison between the rebound tonometer (TONOVET) and the new flattening tonometer (TONO-PEN AVIA) during diurnal curve of intraocular pressure in adult rabbits.** 2010. 58f. Thesis (Master in Veterinary Sciences) - Faculty of Veterinary Medicine, Federal University of Rio Grande do Sul, Porto Alegre. 2010.

PERLMANN, E.; RODARTE-ALMEIDA, A. C. da V. Ocular anatomy and physiology - Literature review. **Medvep - Scientific Journal of Veterinary Medicine - Small Animals and Pets**, Paraná, v. 9, n. 30, p. 410 - 419. 2011.

PETERSON, M. E. Diagnosis of hyperadrenocorticism in dogs. **Clin Tech Small Anim Pract,** Amsterdam, v. 22, n. 1, p. 2 - 11. 2007.

PIPPI, N. L.; GONÇALVES, G. F. **Clinical and Surgical Ophthalmology in Dogs and Cats.** São Paulo: Roca, 2009. 248 p.

QUEIROZ, L. L.; ARIZA, P. C.; LIMA, A. M. V.; FIORAVANTI, M. C. S. Hypertensive retinopathy in dogs and cats. **Enciclopédia Bioesfera**, Goiânia, v. 11, n. 22, p. 2507, 2015.

RAHAL, S. C.; BERGAMO, F. M. M.; ISHIY, H. M. Acrylic resin intraocular prosthesis in dogs and cats. **Brazilian Archive of Veterinary Medicine and Zootechnics.** Belo Horizonte, v. 52, n. 4, p. 319 - 324. 2000.

RAMSEY, I.; RISTIC, J. Diagnosis of canine hyperadrenocorticism. In: **Veterinary Clinics of North America: Small Animal Practice**, v. 29, p. 446 - 454. 2007.

REIS, B. V. G. M. **Clinical aspects of Cushing's syndrome in dogs - literature review**. Recife, 2009, 39f. Post-graduation course conclusion work, Universidade Federal Rural do Semi-Árido.

REUSCH, C. E.; SCHELLENBERG, S.; WENGER, M. Endocrine hypertension in small animals. **Vet Clin Small Anim,** Philadelphia, v. 40, p. 335 - 352. 2010.

SCARAMPELLA, F. Endocrine Alopecia in the Dog. **Veterinary Focus**, France, v. 21, n. 1, p. 40 - 46. 2011.

SILVA, R. F. G. **Study of twenty cases of hyperadrenocorticism in the dog**. Lisbon, 2013, 56f. Dissertation (Master in Veterinary Medicine) - Faculty of Veterinary Medicine, Lusófona University of Humanities and Technologies.

SLATTER, D. **Fundamentals of veterinary ophthalmology.** 3 ed. São Paulo: Roca, 2005. 686 p.

SMETS, P.; MEYER, E.; MADDENS, B.; DAMINET, S. Cushing's syndrome, glucocorticoids and the kidney. **General and comparative endocrinology**, Colorado, v. 169, p. 1 - 10. 2010.

STROM, A. R.; HÄSSIG, M.; IBURG, T. M.; SPIESS, B. M. Epidemiology of canine glaucoma presented to University of Zurich from 1995 to 2009. Part 2:secondary glaucoma (217 cases). **Veterinary Ophthalmology**, Malden, v. 14, n. 2, p. 127-132. 2011.

TAODA, T.; HARA, Y.; MASUDA, H.; TESHIMA, T.; NEZU, Y.; TRAMOTO, A. Magnetic resonance imaging assessment of pituitary posterior lobe displacement in dogs with pituitary-dependent hyperadrenocorticism. **J. Vet. Med. Sci**, Japan, v. 73, n. 6, p. 725 - 731. 2011.

TALIERI, I. C.; BRUNELLI, A. P.; ORIÁ, A. P.; LAUS, J. L. Ophthalmic examination in dogs and cats. **Clínica Veterinária**, São Paulo, n.61, p.42-54. 2006.

TEBALDI, M. **Blood pressure in dogs: a review**. São Paulo, 2011, 21f. Course completion work - Faculty of Veterinary Medicine and Zootechny, Universidade Estadual Paulista.

TEIXEIRA, R. B. **Hyperadrenocorticism in dogs - Literature review**. Tuiuti University of Paraná [online]. Available: http://www.utp.br/medicinaveterinaria/jornadaacademica/HIPER_EM_CAES. Html. [Captured on 12 Dec. 2015].

WILKIE, D. A. **Saunders Manual: Small Animal Clinic.** São Paulo: Roca, 2003. 1808 p.

WILLIS, D. A. Ocular hypotensive drugs. **Veterinary Clinics of North America: Small Animal Practice,** Philadelphia, v. 34, n. 3, p. 755-776. 2004.

33

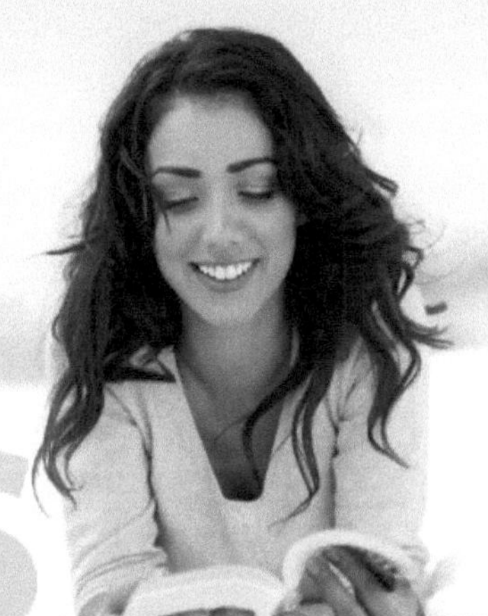

Buy your books fast and straightforward online - at one of world's fastest growing online book stores! Environmentally sound due to Print-on-Demand technologies.

Buy your books online at
www.morebooks.shop

Kaufen Sie Ihre Bücher schnell und unkompliziert online – auf einer der am schnellsten wachsenden Buchhandelsplattformen weltweit! Dank Print-On-Demand umwelt- und ressourcenschonend produziert.

Bücher schneller online kaufen
www.morebooks.shop

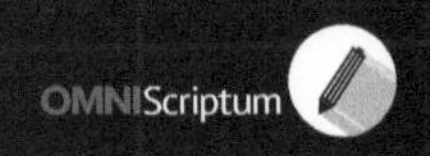

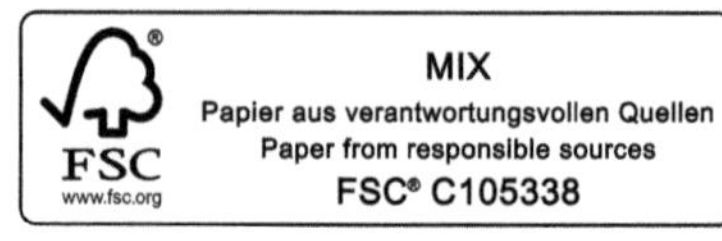

Printed by Books on Demand GmbH, Norderstedt / Germany